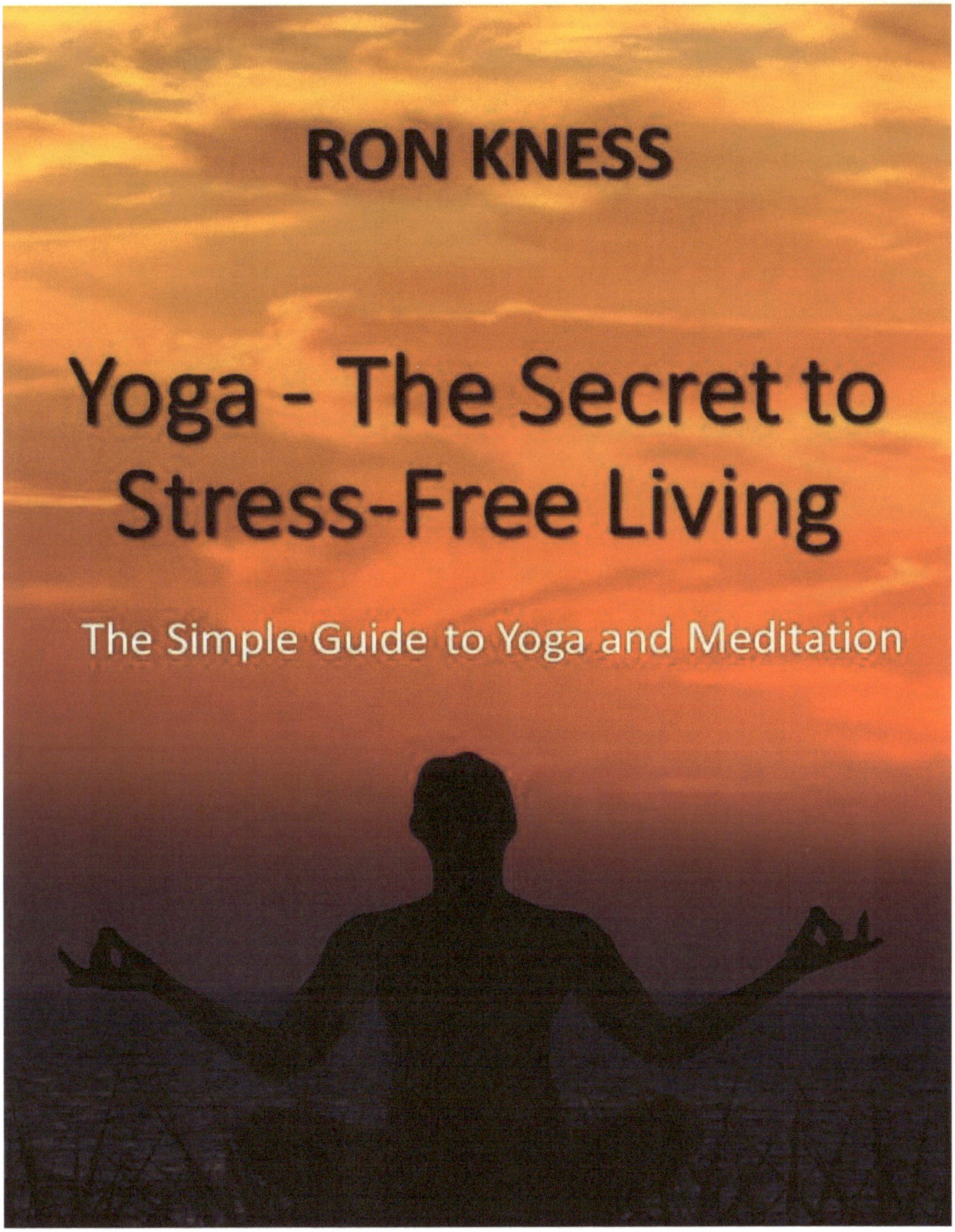

RON KNESS

Yoga - The Secret to Stress-Free Living

The Simple Guide to Yoga and Meditation

Healthy Lifestyle Newsletter.com

(https://healthylifestylenewsletter.com)

Yoga – The Secret to Stress-Free Living

Published by:

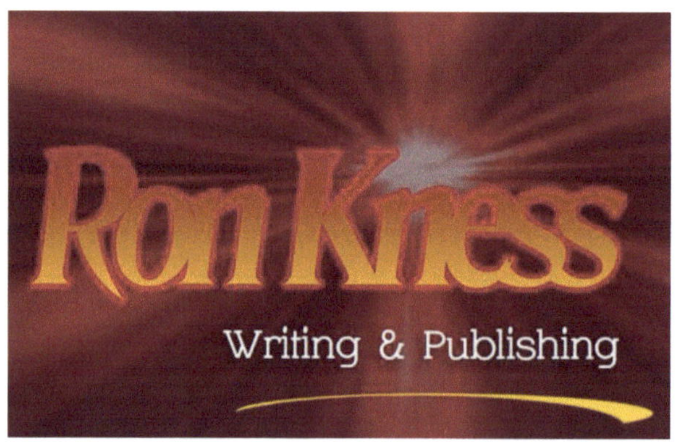

Ron Kness

San Tan Valley, AZ

United States of America

ISBN: 9781792745003

Disclaimer

This publication is protected under the US Copyright Act of 1976 and all other applicable international, federal, state and local laws, and all rights are reserved.

 Please note that much of this publication is based on personal experience and anecdotal evidence. Although the author and publisher have made every reasonable attempt to achieve complete accuracy of the content in this Guide, they assume no responsibility for errors or omissions. Also, you should use this information as you see fit, and at your own risk. Your particular situation may not be exactly suited to the examples illustrated here; in fact, it's likely that they won't be the same, and you should adjust your use of the information and recommendations accordingly.

This publication is for informational purposes only and is not intended as medical advice. Medical advice should always be obtained from a qualified medical professional for any health conditions or symptoms associated with them.

See your healthcare professional before starting any diet, health or exercise program!

Contents

What is Yoga?

Yoga is a physical, mental and spiritual science that originated on the Indian subcontinent over 4,000 years ago. The Sanskrit word "yoga" means concentration or contemplation and is often translated as "union".

It is through the practice of yoga that you can unite mind, body and spirit. Yoga is not just an exercise system, but it is also a philosophy and, if you want it to be, it can become a way of life.

There is no particular religion attached to yoga and people of all faiths practice it. Nor do

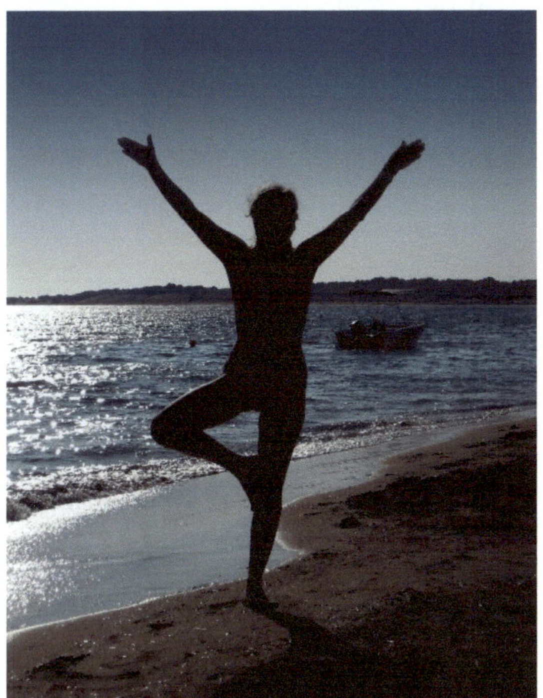

you have to be a particular body type or at a particular fitness level to practice yoga.

Yoga is open to all, which is partly why it has become so popular in the West, although we have adapted and modified the traditional systems of yoga to a style that is more accessible for us.

Western practitioners of yoga have generally kept the basic philosophy and physical poses while not delving too deeply into the more abstract, intellectual aspects which are still considered a part of the practice in India.

The ancient teaching of yoga did not separate mind and body and yoga practice has always included breathing as one of its most important aspects. Newcomers to yoga may, at first, be put off by the emphasis on the spiritual but they quickly come to understand that this is taken in a very wide context.

Yoga is about tapping into our spirit and about believing in things we cannot necessarily see but it is grounded in factual, physical teaching.

In yoga, balance is all - the ultimate aim being to bring about a sense of relaxation and well-being. The yogic view of fitness involves balance and integration, covering all aspects of ourselves and our lives. There are many different styles of yoga with some of the better-known being:

- **Raja** or Royal yoga
- **Karma** yoga or the yoga of destiny
- **Bhakti** or devotional yoga

Yoga – The Secret to Stress-Free Living

- **Mantra** yoga or the yoga of sound
- **Hatha** or physical yoga which can be further subdivided into:
    - Viniyoga
    - Iyengar
    - Astanga Vinyasa
    - Sivananda

Hatha yoga is perhaps one of the most well-known forms of yoga and, if you have taken a yoga class in the past, it is likely that you have come across it. Hatha yoga was specifically designed as an introductory form of yoga and is therefore especially suitable for beginners.

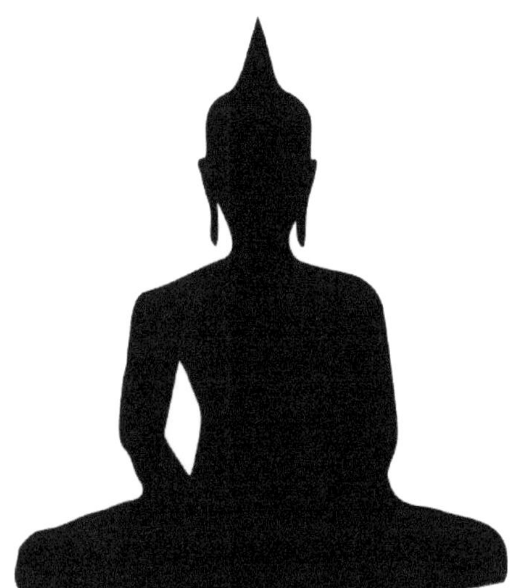

Through practising its techniques, beginners gain control over the mind and body and are therefore able to progress to more complex levels. The exercise sequence you will find later in this book is based upon Sivananda yoga, a particularly gentle form of Hatha yoga.

Raja yoga is often referred to as the king of yogas because the Sanskrit word "raja" means ruler. This classic school of yoga is the yoga of controlling the mind and of meditation. When you see pictures of Buddha meditating, he is practising Raja yoga.

While learning Raja yoga, a student progresses from concentration to contemplation and finally to the ultimate stage which is called Samadhi. This is a state of liberation in which consciousness rises above everyday trials and tribulations.

Karma yoga is based on the belief that we should open up to our intuition when calm and quiet so that can understand what actions we need to take in life. The Sanskrit word "karma" means work and destiny. Once we understand what actions to take, we must carry them out selflessly, without aiming for any reward.

This essentially means doing the right thing in the circumstances no matter how uncomfortable that might be for us. Karma yoga tells its followers to live for the moment and to value the present.

Bhakti yoga is devotional yoga and is particularly appealing to those who are of a religious or spiritual disposition. Bhakti is based upon the concept of adoration, which plays a part in so many major religions. It is a very personal form of yoga through which you can achieve a higher state of consciousness. Many of its practitioners focus upon their particular concept of God when meditating.

Yoga – The Secret to Stress-Free Living

Mantra yoga is the form practised by Tibetan monks. The chanting of mantras raises consciousness and is central to Tibetan meditation. Chanting has always been a natural and pleasurable human activity and is one way of expressing emotion as well as gaining focus. You can learn more about mantras later in this book.

All forms of yoga, in spite of their subtle differences, are based upon the fundamental principle of breath. Specifically, the air and the energy contained within breath which, in yoga terms, is referred to as "prana" or life force. Learning to breathe properly is vital to the successful practice of yoga as, once this is mastered, it means you can also control your thoughts and emotions and hence reduce your stress level.

The physical positions in yoga are referred to as "asanas". These are designed to stretch and tone your muscles, to increase your flexibility, to stimulate your glands and organs and ultimately to relax your entire body.

The word "asana" means to be present and this is another fundamental quality you need to bring to your yoga practice. The fluidity and grace gained through practising the asanas will, in turn, lead to a greater sense of ease and self-confidence when dealing with daily life.

Meditation is also considered part of yoga practice and is important for the mental and spiritual benefits it brings. In this book you will learn simple methods of meditation which are perfect for beginners and adepts alike.

These meditations will allow you to get in touch with the inner quiet of your spirit, thereby nourishing and protecting it from stress.

In our hectic daily lives, yoga and meditation provide a real chance to de-stress and remove ourselves to a safer, quieter place. This is why yoga continues to grow in popularity despite being such an ancient practice and it is also why many health professionals recommend it to help tackle all sorts of ills associated with excessive chronic stress ranging from high blood pressure to osteoporosis.

Young or old, flexible or not so flexible, yoga is the perfect way to gain true holistic fitness and simplify your life.

The Benefits of Yoga

Yoga has been described as the heart of healing and it provides a uniquely harmonising effect for the entire body.

Thanks to its emphasis on deep, rhythmic and effective breathing, yoga not only increases

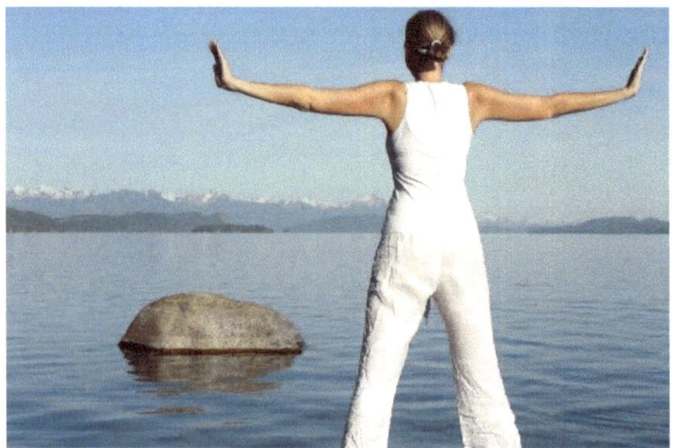

lung capacity and oxygenation of the brain but also the flow of electromagnetic energy which is generated by the heart and transported around the body by the nervous system.

While poor breathing may not always be at the root of depression, it is a fact that people who are depressed or who are suffering from some other kind of mood disorder tend to breathe shallowly and irregularly. By emphasizing effective breathing, yoga can have a very positive effect on the mind as well as the body.

Electrocardiograms have shown the damage to the heart caused by stress and negative thinking and have also demonstrated the healing process that can be brought about by a lessening of stress and more positive thinking.

Yoga also addresses the complaints caused by stress such as tension headaches and hyperventilation. Although it can take long and dedicated practice of yoga to reverse the damage caused by stress and neglect, even complete yoga beginners will soon see an improvement in body function, mental outlook and an immediate decrease in stress to prevent further heart damage in the first place.

Thanks to its emphasis on balanced stretching, yoga can help prevent and ease any number of painful conditions caused by overuse of joints and limbs. These include injuries ranging from hamstring and other sports injuries to conditions such as a frozen shoulder.

Yoga has also been proven to help maintain bone density and to encourage the healthy movement of joints. Better posture, reduced back pain, improved digestion, greater suppleness, clearer sinuses, better balance and improved muscle and skin tone are some of the other benefits of yoga.

Yoga for Inner Peace

One of the benefits of yoga most sought after by Western practitioners is the sense of inner peace that it creates. This can best be described as the marvellous sensation of simply *being* rather than *doing* all the time.

This represents a kind of mini-vacation from the pressures of our hectic daily lives and, interestingly, is a result of the total concentration that yoga trains us to achieve.

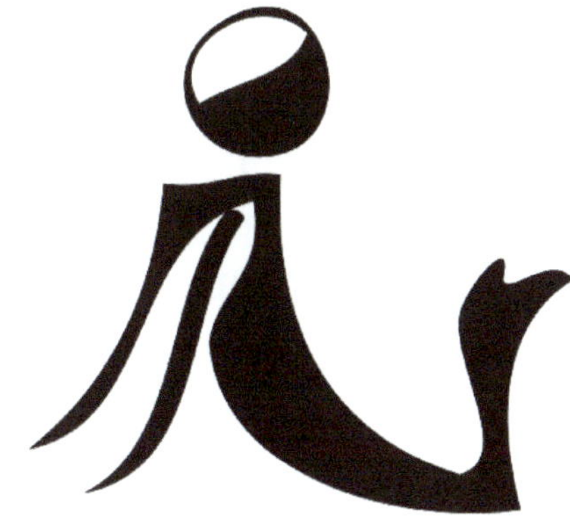

The majority of yoga consists of practising the asanas - originally a variety of sitting positions in which yogis meditated.

Nowadays these have developed to include thousands of other postures all of which, when carried out correctly, free up our breathing and energy. This, in turn, supports our brain function, increasing our capacity to think clearly and to concentrate.

Yoga works with the natural rhythms of the body to help create that sense of inner peace that so many of us crave. By balancing and harmonising the body through correct breathing, yoga can help combat the symptoms of stress, including tension, tiredness, irritability and headaches.

In doing so, yoga helps to foster and maintain the state of inner peace that, in turn, helps us to deal with and manage stress.

Yoga and Healing

Yoga brings us the combined benefits of proper breathing, the asanas and meditation which together form a powerful healing force. Yogis believe that controlled respiration coupled with a focus on a part of the body which is diseased or injured in some way will result in the restoration of the natural functioning of energy or prana in that part of the body.

Complete relaxation forms an important part of Hatha yoga as it eliminates stress and tension that block the flow of prana. Yogis believe that it is the blockage of prana which results in disease.

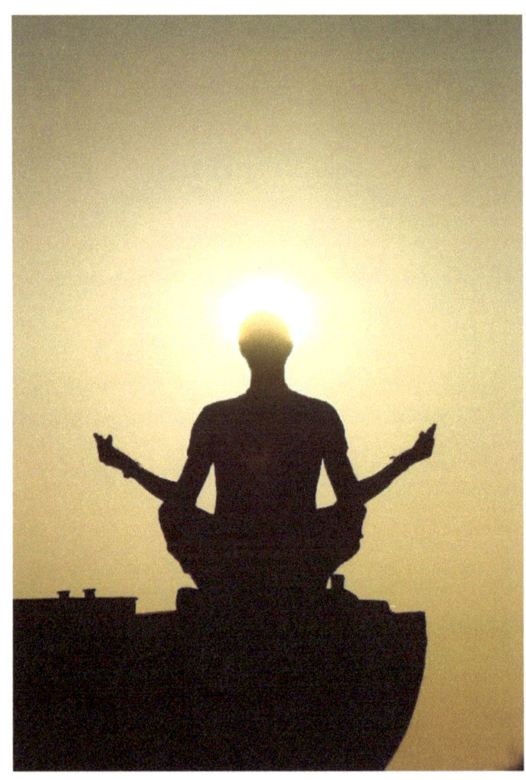

Allowing it to flow more freely through relaxation is considered to be a form of preventative medicine.

Relaxation also leads to a more balanced outlook which, in turn, helps prevent the stress that causes so many of our ills.

There is documented evidence that the release of energy associated with yoga can even help sprains and fractures to heal. This is because a fracture causes an imbalance of energy in the particular part of the body that is affected. Yogis believe that yogic breathing and visualization combined can help restore the flow of energy in the affected area.

Yoga places a lot of emphasis on the importance of visualization to stimulate the body's systems and therefore to help heal them.

Visualization is believed to be so beneficial in easing mental and physical tension that it is often taught to sufferers of particular diseases, most famously cancer. Meditation techniques have also been taught to cancer sufferers to help treat their symptoms.

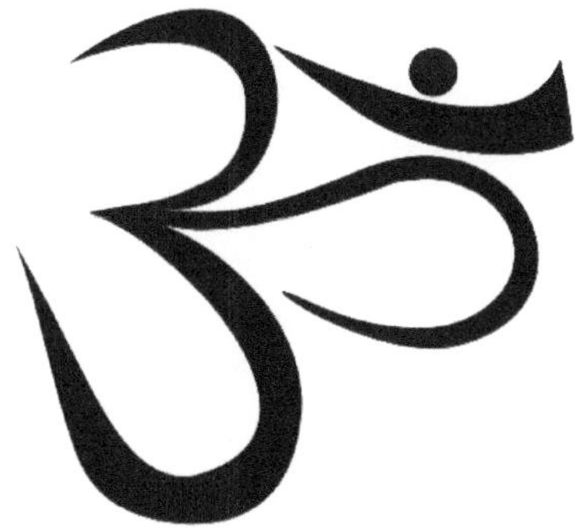

Yoga – The Secret to Stress-Free Living

Breathing

Breathing is, as we know, essential to life. In Sanskrit the word for life and breath is exactly the same and it is one you have already come across: prana.

We need to breathe in order to live and, in order to practice yoga or meditation, we need to learn how to breathe correctly. You can do this by following these easy steps:

- Find a quiet, comfortable place where you can sit with your legs crossed in front of you. If you wish, you can sit in Lotus position, the classic seated asana where each foot rests on the opposite thigh.
- Sit up straight and allow your shoulders to relax away from your ears. Tilt your chin slightly towards your chest.
- Put one hand on your navel and place the other on your lower back so that you can feel your belly expanding as you inhale.
- Keeping your lower jaw relaxed and your mouth closed, breathe in and out slowly through your nose. Imagine that your abdomen is a balloon and that you are filling and then deflating it with every breath.
- Try to picture the lower part of your lungs and imagine yourself filling them up from the bottom to the top. Make sure that your inhalation is long, deep and expansive and that your exhalation is slow and complete.
- When you have practised this for a few minutes, relax, stand up and shake out. Repeat every day for a week and you will find that not only will your have energy increased but also your concentration and your ability to stay calm in stressful situations.

Don't get frustrated if, at first, you can't seem to get this sequence right. Yoga is all about practice and does not demand or expect perfection.

Most people will find that, to start with, they seem to have a fairly small lung capacity and this is usually due to lack of correct use. The more you practice this, deepening your breath and expanding your lungs, you will find that your lung capacity grows enormously over time.

By breathing in deeply enough to draw air into the lower part of your lungs, you get seven times the oxygen you would normally have taken in through general breathing.

In yoga, there are several different forms of breathing, the most well-known being:

- Ujayii or the Special Yogic Breath

- The Energizing Breath
- The Cooling Breath
- The Balancing Breath
- Ujjayi or the Special Yogic Breath

Ujjayi is a method of breathing that is specific to yoga. It involves breathing in and out through the nose while permitting the breath to create a gentle sound at the back of the throat.

Some people liken this method of breathing to the way that Darth Vader breathes in Star Wars. It can also be compared to the way you breathe through your mouth when fogging up a mirror except that it is done through the nose.

Although this form of breathing feels and sounds very strange at first, you will find that the more you do it, the more you focus on the rhythm of your breath and on the sensation of the air filling your body.   The Ujjayi breath is all about breathing in life force, or prana, so that we can both practice yoga and live in a more complete, energised way.

The Energizing Breath

The Energizing Breath also known as the Breath of Fire and is considered in ancient Indian philosophy to cure many illnesses.

The Energizing Breath is perfect for when you're tired and need a quick energy boost or for when you simply need to clear your mind. To practice the Energizing Breath follow these steps:

- Sit with your legs crossed and place both hands on your lower abdomen so that you can feel what happens with your breath.
- Breathe in through your nose, keeping the breath long and deep, feeling your belly filling up. Exhale in the same fashion, feeling your belly deflating as if it were a balloon. Do this 3 to 5 times.
- After the last long inhalation, perform 10 fast exhalations, allowing yourself a short inhalation between each exhalation. Repeat 2 to 3 times.

If you begin to feel dizzy while practising the Energizing Breath, simply curl forward, bringing your head down to your knees and taking a few long, deep breaths.

The Energizing Breath does require some practice so do not get frustrated if at first you are not able to get it right.

Yoga – The Secret to Stress-Free Living

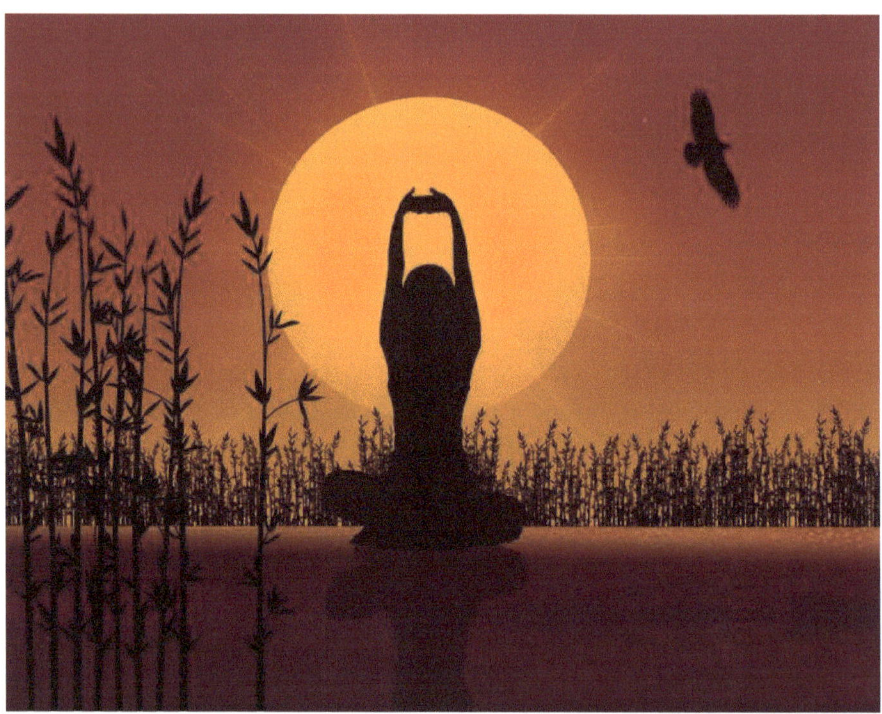

The Cooling Breath

The Cooling Breath slows down your heart rate allowing you to center and calm yourself while regaining your focus. To practice the Cooling Breath follow these steps:

- Curl your tongue and stick it out a little so that when you breathe in it is as if you're sucking the air in through a straw. Now inhale through your mouth.
- Slowly and gently exhale through your nose. Repeat 10 to 15 times.

The Balancing Breath

The Balancing Breath is a technique that has been used by yogis for many hundreds of years to help balance and center both mind and body. To practice the Balancing Breath follow these steps:

- Sit straight with your legs crossed.
- Using your right hand, place your thumb on your right nostril and your ring finger on your left nostril, curling your other fingers into your palm.
- Close the right nostril with your thumb and breathe in through your left nostril for a count of five.
- Now close the left nostril and breathe out through your right nostril for a count of five.

Yoga – The Secret to Stress-Free Living

- Alternate once more and breathe in through the right nostril for a count of five.
- Repeat through the left nostril, exhaling for a count of five and carry on in this way for anything up to 15 minutes.

Meditation

There are many different meditation methods and the key is to choose one that suits you as an individual.

We all concentrate in different ways, some people concentrating more easily on sound while others prefer to focus on an image or on their breathing.

Meditation is all about being at one with yourself in silence and stillness. It is therefore essential choose the meditation method that easily allows you to achieve this state.

Here are three simple meditation methods which are suitable for both complete beginners and those who have more practice.

As with all yoga practice, meditation improves with repetition and experience. If at first you find your mind wandering, simply allow whatever thoughts pop up to float across and then out of your mind without paying them too much attention.

As you become more skilled at meditation, you will no longer find stray thoughts intrusive. Just relax and give yourself to the experience knowing that you will gain a great deal from it, especially if you make it a regular practice.

Breathing Meditation

Classical yoga favors focusing on the breath as a method of meditation. Our breath is considered to be our own, natural mantra and through it we can tune into the silence within ourselves. To practice a breathing meditation, follow the steps below:

- Choose a cushion or blanket as your meditation cushion. If you choose a blanket, fold it up once or twice so that it is comfortable to sit on. Now pick a quiet spot where you will be undisturbed.
- Sit with your legs crossed or in the Lotus position, where each foot is placed on top of the opposite thigh rather than underneath.
- Sit up straight and allow your chin and shoulders to relax just as you did when you were breathing. Close your eyes.
- Relax and breathe in and out naturally.
- Now begin to slow your breath, inhaling to a count of three and exhaling to a count of three, breathing in through the nose and out through your mouth.

- Try to establish a flowing rhythm, neither forcing nor pushing the breath but simply allowing it to be.
- Bring all your attention to your breath, emptying your mind of any extraneous thoughts.
- If any thoughts do pop into your head, simply accept them and then exhale them on the out-breath.
- Be careful not to over breathe or you will start to feel dizzy. Keep your shoulders, head and neck relaxed.
- When you are ready, bring your breathing back to its regular rhythm, open your eyes and slowly become aware of your surroundings.
- Take your time when standing up, stretch out and carry on with your day or evening, enjoying the profound sense of calm and relaxation that you have gained from your meditation.

Visual Meditation

Many of us find it easier to meditate when we are focusing on a particular image or object.

One particularly popular method is to focus on a candle flame. To practice this candle meditation, follow the steps below:

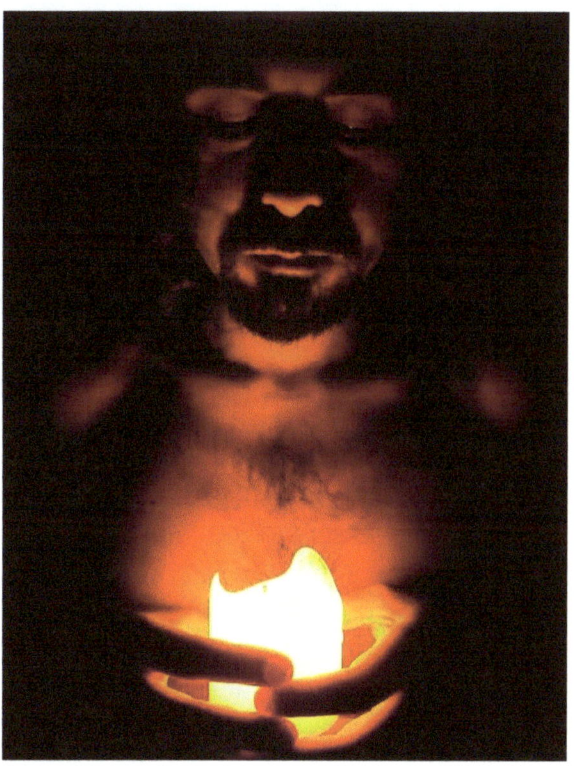

- Choose a cushion or blanket as your meditation cushion. If you choose a blanket, fold it up once or twice so that it is comfortable to sit on. Now pick a quiet spot where you will be undisturbed.
- Sit with your legs crossed or in the Lotus position, where each thigh is placed on top of the opposite thigh rather than underneath.
- Place a candle in an appropriate holder in a position where you can easily gaze at it. It is better to place it below eye level so that you are gazing down at it without having to tilt your head or chin in a strained manner.
- Take a few moments to center yourself before lighting the candle.
- Now sit up straight and allow your chin and shoulders to relax just as you did when you were breathing.

Yoga – The Secret to Stress-Free Living

- Bring your focus to the candle flame, trying not to stare too hard at it but rather to feel as if your gaze is melding with the flame.
- Allow your breathing to slow to a rhythmic intake and exhalation but do not force it or concentrate too hard on it.
- Continue to gaze at the candle flame as you slowly allow your mind to empty. If thoughts should pop into your head, simply allow them to drift through and away.
- Feel yourself becoming at one with the flame, allowing its energy to flow through you and your energy to flow through it.
- If you become distracted, gently bring yourself back to your meditation. When you are ready, slowly bring your awareness back to your surroundings, blow out the candle and stretch, enjoying the sense of calm and focus that you can carry with you.

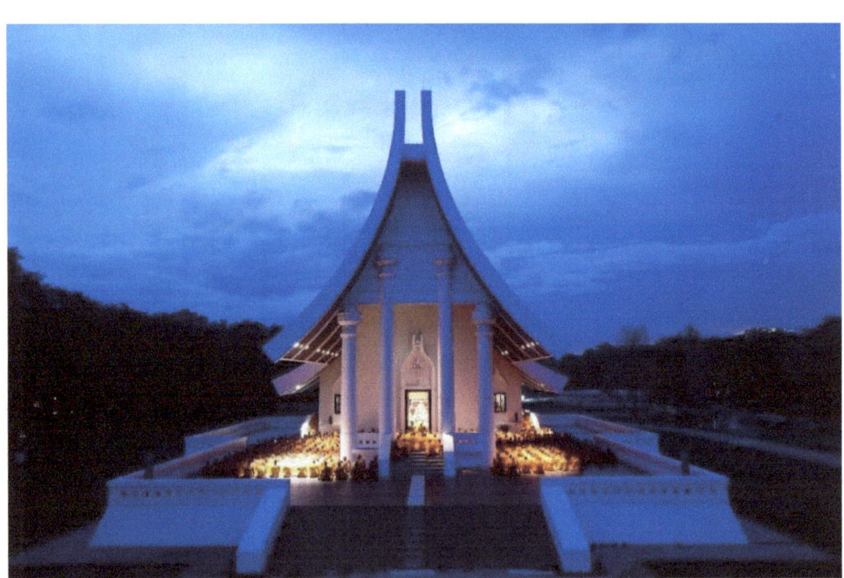

Mandalas and Yantras

Where mantras are used as a form of sound meditation (see below), yantras and mandalas are used as an aid to visual meditation. A yantra is a mystical symbol of cosmic energy and power.

Typically, it takes the form of a geometric diagram consisting of circles, triangles, Lotus petals and sometimes gods or goddesses.

If you are using a yantra as an aid to meditation, you focus on the central point or 'bindu' which is considered to be the sacred symbol of the universe. When using a yantra you are supposed to look beyond the visual patterns and into its structure and essence. Your understanding of a particular yantra grows over time.

Yoga – The Secret to Stress-Free Living

A mandala is more pictorial than a yantra and consists of circular arrangements of patterns and icons. Both mandalas and yantras influenced the structure and layout of Hindu and Buddhist temples.

Similar structural arrangements are found at other sacred sites, including England's Stonehenge and the Mayan pyramids in Mexico.

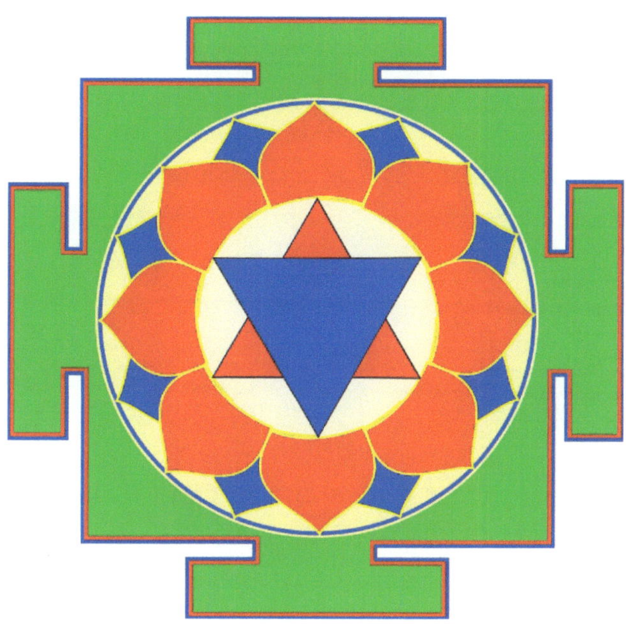

Mantra Meditation

A mantra meditation uses sound to instil and deepen focus. A mantra is simply something that your mind projects - it can be a picture, a color, a word, a thought, a feeling or an affirmation. You may have heard traditional Sanskrit mantras used in Buddhist chants.

You don't have to use these but instead can use your own phrase which can be something as simple as: 'I am calm and centered'. There are ideas for mantras later on in this chapter.

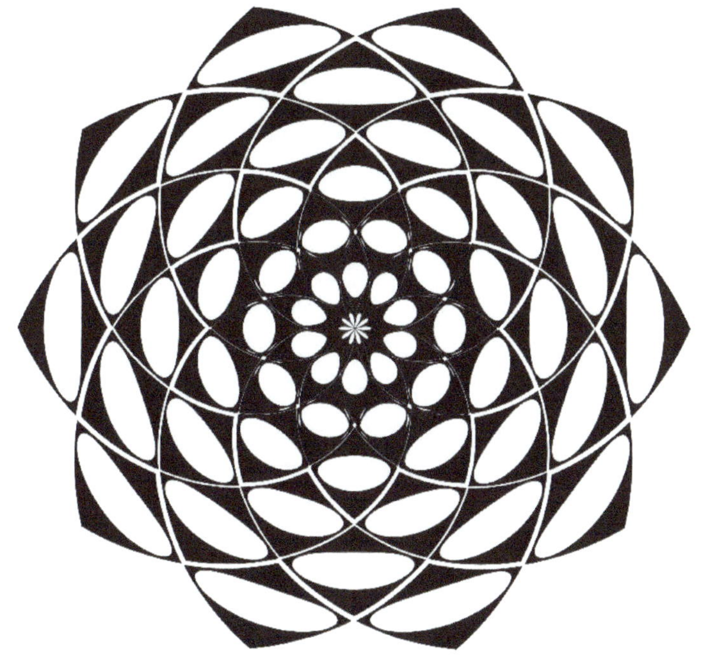

Yoga – The Secret to Stress-Free Living

To practice a mantra meditation, follow the steps below:

- Choose a cushion or blanket as your meditation cushion. If you choose a blanket, fold it up once or twice so that it is comfortable to sit on. Now pick a quiet spot where you will be undisturbed.
- Sit with your legs crossed or in the Lotus position, where each foot is placed on top of the opposite thigh rather than underneath.
- Sit up straight and allow your chin and shoulders to relax just as you did when you were breathing. Close your eyes.
- Relax and breathe in and out naturally.
- Start to focus your attention on the center of your forehead which is a place commonly known as your third eye or sixth chakra.
- Now place your palms together at chest height breathe in deeply and, on the exhalation, recite out loud or to yourself a mantra.
- Whatever mantra you choose, repeat it three times and then take a few minutes to simply relax and breathe.

Some Ideas for Mantras

As you already know, a mantra can be almost anything you choose although most people prefer some kind of chant. Many traditional mantras are written in Sanskrit while others are Buddhist chants.

If you would like to try one of these traditional mantras, here are some suggestions:

- **Ong Namo (pronounced Nah-mo) Guru Dev Namo** - this means, "I honor the teacher within my own being."
- **Om Namah Shivaya** – means the same as above but from the Hindu culture.
- **Ad Guray Nameh** (Ahd Gu-ray Na-may)
- **Jugad Guray Nameh** (Ju-god Gu-ray Na-may)
- **Sat Guray Nameh** (Sat Gu-ray Na-may)
- **Siri Guru Dev Nameh** (Si-ri Gu-ru De-Vay Na-may) This means: "I bow to the wisdom of the universe and to the wisdom of my own being."
- **Om** or **Aum** - perhaps one of the most famous mantras of all, this is considered to be the sound of the universe in perfect harmony. Chanted as a mantra, it enables you to tune into the universal flow of all life. The physical symbol of "om" or "aum" is the conch shell and it is believed to embody the highest reaches of subtle sound.

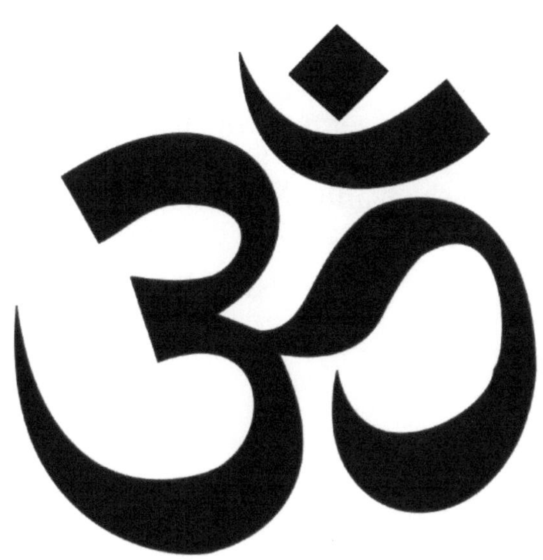

The Chakras

You have already learned about the yoga concept of life force or energy otherwise known as prana. We all have seven energy centers which are known as "chakras".

The work "chakra" means wheel and it may help you to visualize each center as a vortex spinning with energy. The chakras start at the base of the spine, finishing at the top of the head.

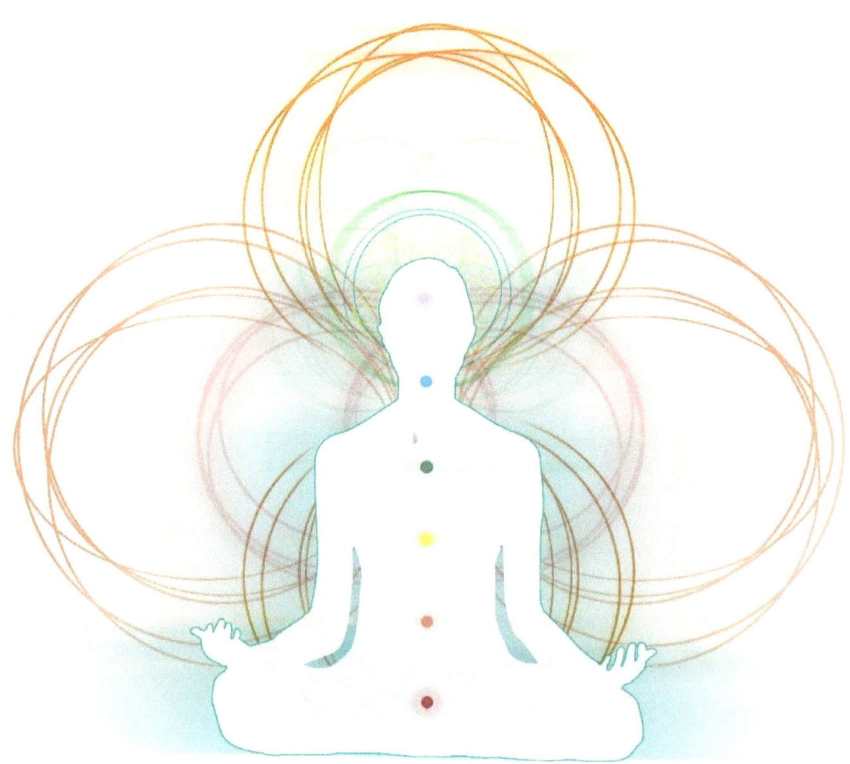

Yoga – The Secret to Stress-Free Living

Each chakra corresponds to a different point on the body. The traditional chakra system was designed to help yogis remember the form of the universe. Although it is hard for us to truly understand the yoga concept of prana, particularly because it is invisible, we can appreciate that when our energy is balanced we operate at our best.

As the chakras are centers of energy, it follows that when they are imbalanced we may feel unwell or simply a little 'off.'

Here is a list of the chakras and how each relates to our needs:

1. **The first or root chakra** - is symbolized by the color red and is located at the base of the spine. This chakra relates to our most basic need to survive.
2. **The second chakra** - is symbolized by the color orange and is located beneath the navel. This chakra relates to creativity, sexuality, self- esteem and self-acceptance.
3. **The third chakra** - is symbolized by the color yellow and is located at the solar plexus. This chakra relates to power, growth and control.
4. **The fourth chakra** - is symbolized by the color green and is located at the heart. This chakra relates to the way we feel and express love and compassion.
5. **The fifth chakra** - is symbolized by the color blue and is located at the throat. This chakra relates to communication, truth and understanding.

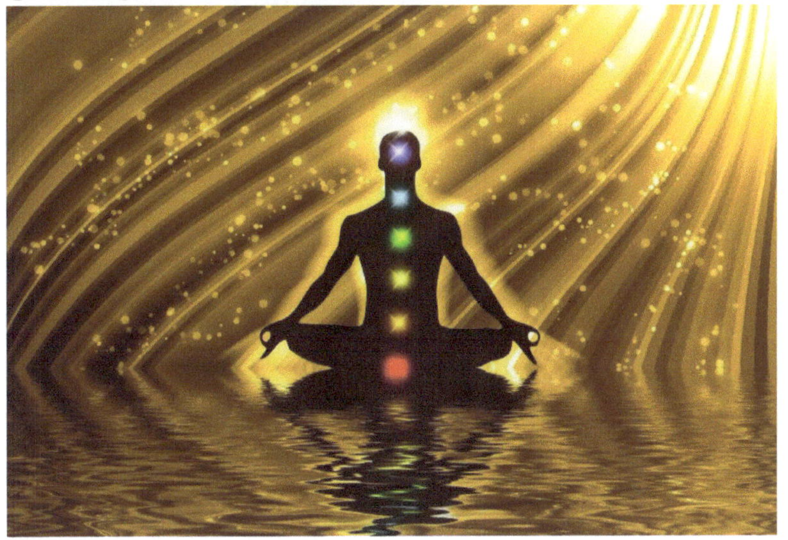

6. **The sixth chakra** - is symbolized by the color indigo and is located at the third eye, slightly above and between the eyebrows. This chakra relates to intuition and wisdom.
7. **The seventh chakra** - is symbolized by the color violet and is located at the crown of the head. This chakra relates to our connection to the universe and self-realization.

When we are practising proper breathing we move prana through the body, which allows energy to flow freely. By awakening the chakras through yoga, you can draw in the Earth's energy as you breathe.

Yoga – The Secret to Stress-Free Living

Testing the Chakras

You can test how well this works by carrying out the exercise below. You will need to do this with the help of another person:

- Stand with your feet a few inches apart and hold your right arm out to the side with your fist clenched so that your muscles tense.
- Your partner now stands behind you, pressing down on one or more of the muscles in your extended arm so that they can check strength and tone.
- Keeping your right arm extended and your fist clenched, press your left hand into your abdomen just above the navel, curling in your fingers to do so. Your partner should now press down again on your right arm and will be able to feel that it is considerably weaker.
- Now let both arms drop to your sides and breathe in and out deeply at least 10 times. Try to keep your chest and abdomen as still as possible while imagining that you are inflating your lungs to their fullest as if they were balloons. For a reminder of how to do this, turn back to the section on breathing.
- Once you have completed your breathing exercise, extend your right arm again, clenching your fist to tense the muscles. Ask your partner to press down on the arm again and they should find that it is a lot stronger.
- Repeat steps one and two but, this time, press the fingers of your left hand into the base of your breastbone or sternum. You should find that, this time, your right arm remains strong.

Kundalini

Kundalini is the vast reserve of energy that lies dormant at the base of the spine until it has awakened by something such as yoga. Kundalini is translated as "Serpent Power" and is symbolised by a snake.

While the practice of yoga asanas and breathing frees up the body's energy in a controlled way, attempting to release kundalini energy should only be attempted on the expert guidance.

Choosing the Right Form of Yoga

Before trying out different methods of yoga, it is a good idea to identify your body type. Classical Indian medicine, known as Ayurveda, classifies body types through 'doshas.'

These doshas consist of air, otherwise known as Vata, fire or Pitta and earth or Kapha. It is through balancing these three qualities that we maintain our health.

Practitioners of Indian medicine diagnose patients as being predominantly one dosha, or more usually two. Understanding our doshas can help us to make the right choices when it comes to diet, environment and exercise.

Coffee, for example, may act as a beneficial stimulant for someone who is predominantly Kapha while for a predominantly Vata type, it could literally send them spinning.

Here is a general outline of the doshas but bear in mind that this is merely a tiny part of what is a vast area of study. Read through the descriptions and decide which dosha is dominant for you so that you can then choose the appropriate method of yoga.

Vata

- Element: Air
- Controls: Bodily movement
- Characteristics: Light, slender build. Is enthusiastic and excitable although sometimes restless. Tends to have bursts of energy, moving quickly. Can be a worrier and tends to suffer from changeable moods. Quick to learn but may have problems focusing. Irregular appetite and can be prone to digestive problems.
- Suggested method of yoga: Viniyoga or Sivananda, both of which are soothing and grounding. Other methods need to be taken gently. This type needs a lot of rest and relaxation.
- When balanced: A Vata type is happy, imaginative, enthusiastic and alert.

Pitta

- Element: Fire
- Controls: Metabolism and digestion.
- Characteristics: Courageous, articulate, intelligent, competitive, can anger easily. Tends to be of medium build and stamina. Loves a challenge and has a sharp intellect.

Yoga – The Secret to Stress-Free Living

- Suggested method of yoga: This type needs calming and all methods of yoga are beneficial. Might be particularly drawn to Astanga because of the challenge but needs to practice it calmly and with gentle breathing. Needs to balance rest and exercise as this type has a sensitive constitution.
- When balanced: A Pitta type is warm, confident, emotional and content.

Kapha

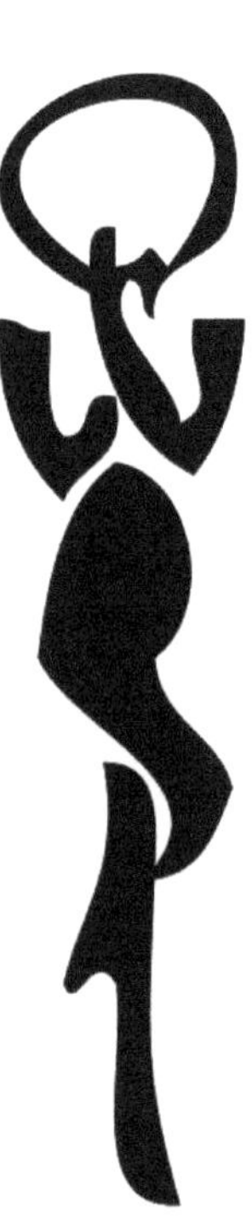

- Element: Earth
- Controls: Bodily structure
- Characteristics: Can be lazy and has a tendency towards obesity. Has a slow digestion and steady energy. Tends to be tranquil and a heavy sleeper. Is affectionate and forgiving while possessing a solid, powerful build.
- Suggested method of yoga: Needs to be energized so both Astanga and Iyengar yoga are ideal. Needs regular, demanding exercise.
- When balanced: Kapha is relaxed, affectionate and calm.
- To be healthy and balanced, we need the qualities of all three doshas. Ayurvedic practitioners prescribe daily Sun salutations followed by 15 minutes of yoga in order to achieve balance and harmony. The yoga should always include six ways of stretching:
    - A forward bend
    - A back bend
    - A side stretch
    - A twist
    - A balance
    - An inversion such as a headstand or a shoulder stand

All of these should be performed with the correct breathing.

Yoga for Particular Groups of People

Yoga for Complete Beginners

If you are a complete yoga beginner, you should try any style you find attractive, bearing in mind your predominant dosha. It is important that you find a teacher to whom you can relate and who inspires you to further your yoga practice.

Iyengar yoga offers an excellent introduction to correct alignment of the body while, on the other hand, Sivananda yoga is a gentle introduction and sets out a clearly defined yoga lifestyle while not emphasizing alignment at all.

Astanga yoga is very physical while Viniyoga takes a personal approach and is profoundly nurturing. Each of these styles will be taught in different ways by different teachers. As you can see, you therefore need to explore to find a style and class that is right for you.

If you prefer, you can simply start with the yoga sequence taught in this book and practice that until you feel you wish to progress some more. Even then, you can simply study more advanced material either via books or DVDs or on the Internet.

Some people prefer the sense of community created by a yoga class while others are content with personal practice. As with all yoga, choose what is right for you.

Yoga for Kids

Yoga is a superb choice for children as the earlier you start to practice in life, the better.

Yoga keeps our spines free and our bodies flexible so is an excellent habit to instill in kids although it is important that it is taught in a fun and creative way.

Many yoga poses appeal visually to children because they are named after animals and nature and learning them stimulates the imagination. Yoga is also an excellent way to help children relax and is therefore particularly suitable for poor sleepers.

The more advanced poses, such as headstands, should not be taught until a child has reached the age of 14 as otherwise they can interfere with bone formation and hormonal changes. Yoga is excellent for teenagers as it helps to calm and to instil self-confidence.

Astanga Vinyasa yoga is particularly recommended after puberty as its dynamic, constant, flowing sequence provides a great exercise routine for a growing body.

Yoga – The Secret to Stress-Free Living

Children have the advantage over adults in that they are less self-conscious and more open to learning. They have less fear about trying new things and yoga helps them to harness their energy.

They are best off learning yoga on a physical level at first, progressing to the more mental and spiritual aspects in their late teens.

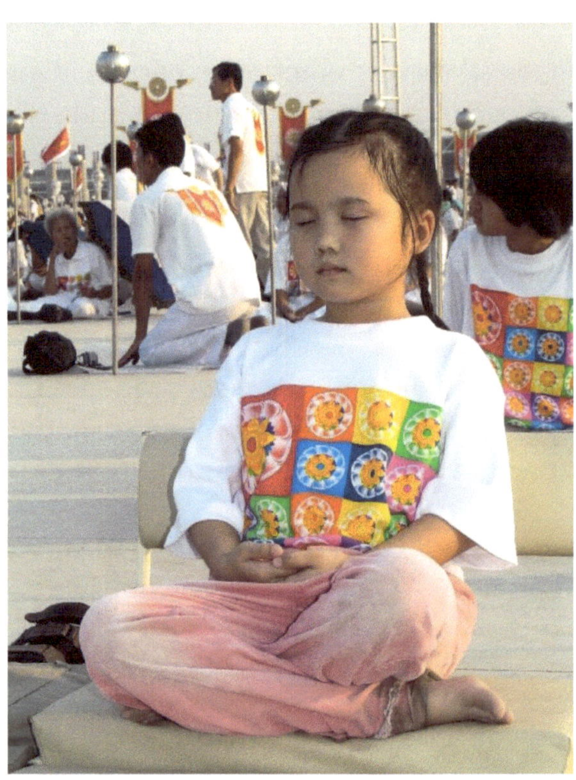

Yoga for Seniors

Sivananda yoga is very gentle and therefore ideal for seniors while Iyengar and Astanga yoga help to stimulate both body and mind and prevent the faculties from slowing.

An alert mind helps to keep the body young and people of all ages need stimulation.

Yoga is an excellent practice for seniors with particular needs and disabilities because it is endlessly adaptable.

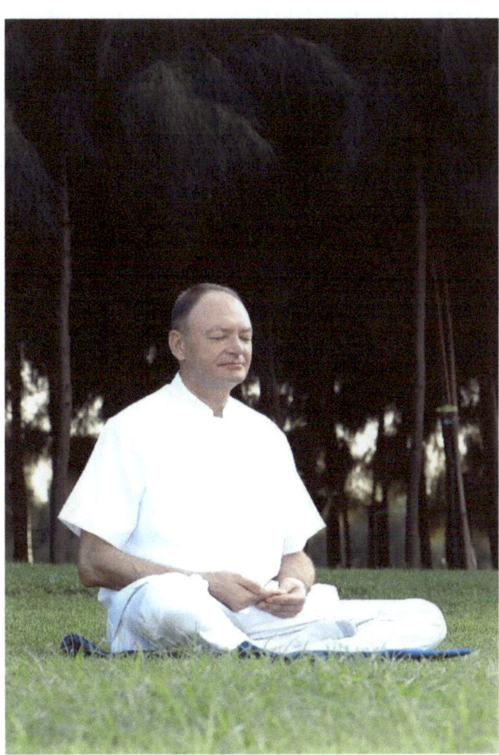

Yoga for Particular Conditions

Yoga for Depression

Depression has been defined as 'the separation from self' which leads to the alienation and isolation so commonly experienced by sufferers. Yoga helps us to harmonise and integrate with ourselves, bringing us back to who we truly are and is therefore extremely helpful in cases of depression.

The breathing practices employed in yoga also work subtly to clear negativity and to bring about acceptance by helping a depressed person breathe through the mental pain.

More vigorous forms of yoga, such as Astanga, stimulate the endorphin release associated with cardiovascular exercise which also helps to cut through depression.

Astanga yoga has been found to be particularly helpful for people coming off anti-depressants as it is both healing and empowering, getting rid of negative ways of thinking.

Yoga for Particular Injuries

Very gentle yoga is advised in cases of injury and, at all times, should be appropriate to the needs of the injured person.

Even if an injury calls for complete bed rest, you can lie in a way that ensures that your blood is well oxygenated which means a healthier heart and organs. Practising yoga breathing will help to achieve this as will lying in Savasana, otherwise known as the corpse posture.

In cases of muscular injury, you can try to work through it physically provided you know how to distinguish between a healthy level of discomfort and the sort of pain that signals you should stop. Iyengar yoga is often used in remedial classes but is not advised if you are suffering from a fever, when you should rest.

It is important to decide what is appropriate according to the particular injury and, in most forms of yoga, an individual program will be prescribed. If you are in any doubt, you should seek out a specialist remedial class.

Yoga for Addiction

Yoga can be very helpful to people coming off drugs and alcohol and there are a number of detox programs that teach it. Yoga helps us to think clearly about ourselves and to remain centered and calm, all of which are highly beneficial when combating addiction.

Meditation practice, in particular, can help address the neurosis that often lies at the heart of an addictive personality.

Yoga to Lose Weight

Astanga yoga is excellent for losing weight and toning up if you are overweight but reasonably fit. If you are overweight and unfit, is a good idea begin with another style and work up to Astanga later to build up your fitness and stamina.

Iyengar is another form that helps to shed weight thanks to its rigorous training, but all yoga styles will help to gradually balance the body and therefore get rid of any excess fat. This works as much on a mental as on a physical level by allowing you to explore what motivates the urge to over eat.

Yoga in Pregnancy

Yoga is excellent both during pregnancy and as a postnatal form of exercise, but it is important to choose a specialist class taught by a suitably qualified teacher. Astanga is not suitable for beginners if you are pregnant but, if you are already a yoga practitioner, you may be able to modify it with a teacher's help.

Yoga for Stress

As all forms of yoga are restorative and balancing, it is an excellent choice if you are stressed. Several forms such as Astanga and Sivananda can be practised in a smooth, flowing style much like Tai Chi. Other, more demanding forms can help dissipate tension and wound up energy.

Sivananda yoga can be highly beneficial to people who need soothing and grounding as sessions start with a headstand and move through to standing asanas, thereby working from the head down.

Balance Is Everything

Yoga is a holistic discipline and balance is therefore central to it. During a yoga session, equal time is allocated to breathing, asanas, relaxation and meditation so that mind, body and brain are given equal importance.

All the asanas complement one another with muscles working in groups rather than individually. An exercise that stretches one muscle group will always be followed by another that works on a complementary group.

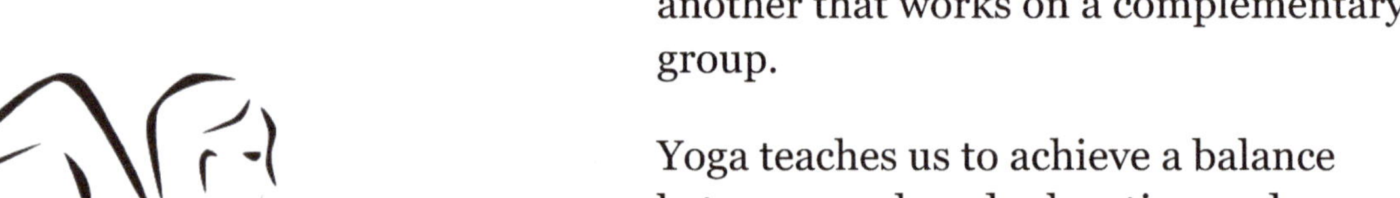

Yoga teaches us to achieve a balance between work and relaxation and a yoga session includes regular pauses for rest in order to dissipate any negative influences.

Yoga asanas may sometimes be difficult, but they invigorate us rather than tiring either mind or body.

Correct breathing helps to maintain the balance between mind and body and is particularly important when practising Hatha yoga.

By learning to apply the principle of balance during our yoga sessions, we can transfer the same skills to everyday life. Yoga teaches us to find contentment within ourselves rather than looking to outside stimuli.

It encourages us to live for the moment and to draw strength from happy events so that every moment is enjoy to its fullest. This also helps to sustain us through more difficult times.

An important difference between other forms of exercise and yoga is that many sports demand that we use the same set of muscles over and over.

Yoga ensures balance by working complementary groups of muscles and by balancing a movement with one that exercises an opposing muscle group.

Yoga – The Secret to Stress-Free Living

Yoga is therefore an excellent choice for athletes as it enables them to exercise muscles they are under using. The resultant increased mobility and flexibility enhances all sports performance.

Preparation for Yoga

To prepare for yoga practice you need to ensure that your body is flexible and that your mind is free. Before a yoga session you need to rid yourself of any tension in either mind or body. There is no one way to do this but here are some suggestions.

It will help if you approach these with an open attitude and a willingness to remain receptive.

Relaxed Breathing

Establishing and encouraging relaxed breathing is an excellent way to approach a yoga session. Here are a couple of exercises which will help you to achieve this:

Mountain or Tadasana

Stand tall with your feet a few inches apart and your arms by your sides, shoulders rolled back and down, backside tucked under. Rotate your hands so that your palms are facing forward. This is Mountain posture or Tadasana.

Take a long in-breath and, as you do so, bring your arms slowly upward until you can rest your hands on the crown of your head, palms touching. Maintain this position as you breathe out slowly.

Take another long in-breath and, as you do so, slowly stretch up your arms, keeping the palms together. Stretch up as high as you can, holding your breath. Maintain this position for a few seconds and then bring your hands back to the crown of your head, still keeping the palms together.

Repeat this 5 to 10 times keeping your breath and movements controlled and coordinated. On your final out-breath bring your arms down to chest level, palms still touching. This is prayer position, or Namaste.

Close your eyes, breathe quietly and repeat the word 'peace' to yourself several times. On another out-breath, separate your palms and bring your arms slowly back down to your sides.

Stretch up once more with palms facing forward while visualizing the peak of a mountain. Do this several times and then relax.

Yoga – The Secret to Stress-Free Living

Flexibility Exercise

Stand tall with your arms by your sides and exhale slowly and deeply. On a long, slow in-breath lift your arms out from your sides, palms facing forward, stretching upwards until your arms are at shoulder level.

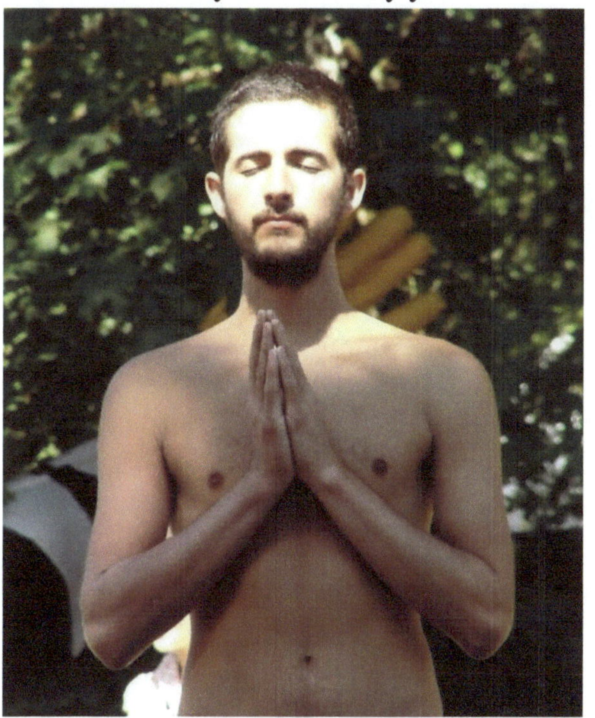

Breathe out once more and stretch your arms and torso forward, leaning from the hips and making sure that you are not bending your back.

Breathe in and, as you do so, swing your arms upwards, bending backwards and allowing your knees to also bend to maintain your balance.

Come back to center and straighten up, breathing out. Still standing straight, take another slow in-breath and, on your next out-breath, perform a sideways bend to your right keeping your hips and shoulders in line.

Breathe in, come back to center, and repeat to the left.

Once back in center, breathe out and slowly allow your head, neck, chest and arms to drop forward from the hips, bending your knees if necessary. Gently swing from side to side several times before slowly coming back up to standing, making sure that your head is the last to come up.

Stand tall with your eyes closed for a few moments, breathing quietly. You will feel calm, focused and refreshed.

Total Body Stretches

Stretching stimulates blood flow to the muscles, releasing tension and improving tone. When coupled with effective breathing, stretching stimulates the flow of energy throughout the entire body which also increases alertness.

The aim when stretching before performing yoga asanas is not to work out but to gently prepare the body for stronger exercise. Stretching can be carried out in any position including sitting or even lying on the floor, as well as standing.

The following two exercises are especially suitable for preparing both mind and body for a yoga session.

Yoga – The Secret to Stress-Free Living

Sitting stretches

Sit tall on a firm, supportive chair and breathe slowly out through your nose. Breathe in and, as you do so, swing your arms upwards so that they are reaching above your head, palms facing forward. Do not hunch your shoulders or strain.

Breathe out sharply through your nose and, as you do so, swing yourself forward so that you are curving your body over your thighs, with your arms flopping either side of your legs, hands resting on the floor. Your chin should be resting somewhere just below your knees.

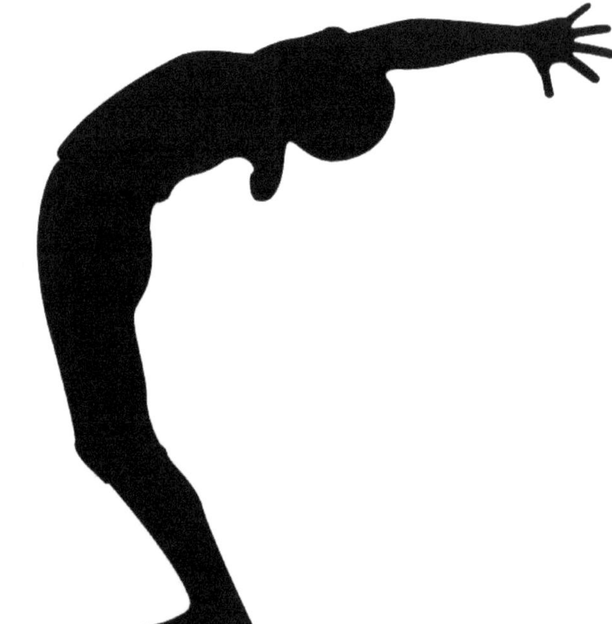

Swing your head gently from side to side to release any tension in the neck and maintain this position for a few seconds.

Come back up to sitting.

Repeat up to 12 times and, when you have finished, sit quietly for a few moments with your eyes closed and your hands resting in your lap.

Standing stretches

Stand tall with your feet about 12 inches apart. Breathe out and, on a long, slow in-breath, swing your arms up above your head thrusting your pelvis forward. Maintain this position for a few seconds.

From here bend forward, swinging your arms down, letting your head drop and your hands rest on the floor. As you do this, breathe out through your mouth making a long 'ha' sound. Bend forward only as far as is comfortable, bending your knees if necessary. Breathe gently in and out through your nose. Maintain this position for about a minute.

On an in-breath, roll back up to standing and push your arms back, palms facing back, allowing yourself to bend back as far as possible without straining. Your lower back will be slightly arched. Maintain this position for about a minute, breathing in and out gently through the nose.

Come back to center, drop your arms to your sides and repeat two or three times.

Yoga – The Secret to Stress-Free Living

Head, Neck and Shoulder Stretch

So many of us carry tension in our head, neck and shoulders, especially as we tend to sit hunched up all day at a desk or in front of a computer. This may at first simply make us feel stiff but, over time, the neck bones can be affected, resulting in chronic pain.

Some people will try to stretch now and again at their desk that this can, in fact, cause even more damage as the body will not be in the right position for this type of movement. Follow the exercises below to stretch the head, neck and shoulders effectively.

Shoulder Shrugging

This exercise is very effective for freeing shoulder muscles and relieving tension. It can be carried out while sitting or standing and, when performed regularly, will relieve chronic stiffness in one or both shoulders.

Sit or stand with your back straight but not stiff, your head centred and balanced, eyes looking forwards and arms by your sides.

Breathe in and, as you do so, shrug both shoulders up towards your ears. Breathe out and let them fall back to their natural position. Repeat three or four times.

Now alternate shoulders, lifting first the left shoulder to the left ear and then the right shoulder to the right ear, breathing in as you lift and out as you drop. Repeat three or four times.

Neck Easer

Perform these exercises whenever your neck feels stiff.

Sit in a firm, supportive chair with your lower back pressing against the chair back, your head centred and balanced, eyes looking forward.

Allow your arms to dangle loosely at your sides. Relax your shoulders.

Breathe in and, on an out-breath, turn your head slowly to the right, finishing the movement as you reach the end of your exhalation.

Maintain this position for a few seconds, breathing in and then, on another out-breath, try to gently turn your head even further to the right. Take a long, slow in-breath.

On your next out-breath, turn your head slowly to the left, finishing the movement as you reach the end of your exhalation.

You should be facing front when you need to breathe in. Take a few long, slow in-breaths and try to relax even further.

Repeat step 2, this time turning your head to the left. Maintain this position for a few seconds, breathing in and then, on another out-breath, try to gently turn your head even further to the left.

Take a long, slow in-breath.

Repeat step 3 until you are facing forward again. Take several long, slow, deep breaths.

On an out-breath, allow your chin to fall gently forwards until it rests on your chest. Breathe in and out slowly and rhythmically, easing your head forward a little more on each out-breath.

On an in-breath, slowly raise your head until you are facing forward. As you begin to breathe out, continue raising it until it is falling gently backwards.

Tighten your jaw, and, breathing in and out, let your head fall back a little further on each out-breath. Remember to keep this gentle. On your final out-breath, slowly bring your head forward once more.

Stretching the Arms, Torso and Legs

There are yoga poses or asanas to exercise practically every muscle in your body but often a short session of yoga will focus on just one area. It is therefore a good idea to spend some of your warm-up time exercising the arms, torso and legs so that you achieve the balance which is essential to yoga practice.

These exercises are particularly good for anyone who spends a lot of time sitting at a desk or in some other kind of static position. Arm stretches are essential for people who spend a lot of time working at the keyboard as they help to prevent and ease RSI (repetitive strain injury).

Following the exercises here will also help you stretch and tone the muscles in your chest, abdomen, limbs, hands and feet.

If you suffer from lower back pain it is a good idea to do these exercises, and indeed any exercise in this book, very gently. You should stop immediately if you experience any pain.

By practising these exercises regularly, you will stretch and realign your lumbar vertebrae which will help to ease and manage lower back pain as well as preventing other serious conditions, such as a slipped disk, from occurring.

Yoga – The Secret to Stress-Free Living

Arm and Hand Stretches

You can perform this either sitting or standing but, in both cases, you need to ensure that you are tall and straight.

Without straining your neck or shoulders, stretch your arms out in front of you at shoulder height, palms facing upwards.

Now bend your arms at the elbow and place your fingertips on your shoulders, right fingertips on right shoulder and left fingertips on left shoulder.

Breathe in and, on your out-breath, snap your arms and hands out in front of you at shoulder height.

Keeping your arms where they are, curl your fingers in to make fists, squeeze tight and then snap your fingers out.

Repeat 10 times and finish by letting your hands and arms go floppy before shaking them gently for a few minutes.

Hip Hula

If you suffer from lower back pain or a slipped disk do not perform this exercise.

Stand tall with your feet shoulder width apart and place your hands on your hips, flexing slightly at your knees.

Keeping your shoulders reasonably still, push your right hip slowly out to the right, then back to center, then left, then forward several times until you are gyrating rhythmically. Repeat once more, this time starting with your left hip.

You can vary this by speeding up, slowing down or by doing this exercise to music. There is no need to focus on your breathing but simply to allow it to follow your movements.

Feet Flexes

Sit tall on the floor with your legs stretched out in front of you, feet a few inches apart. You can place your hands on the floor either side of your hips or slightly behind them if you feel you need support.

Start by trying to wriggle each toe in turn, flexing them forwards and backwards as well as from side to side if possible. Do not manipulate them with your fingers and try to move them independently of each other.

Now bend your right leg and rest the ankle on your left thigh so that your foot is free. Grasp your right foot with your left hand supporting the ball of your foot and rotate it several times in both directions.

Repeat with your left foot resting on your right thigh.

Relaxation Exercises

During any yoga session there will always be pauses for relaxation. These are to allow both body and mind to rest between the asanas. At the end of the session there should be a longer period of relaxation. True relaxation is not achieved by simply allowing the body to flop.

In order to really relax, the body needs to be in a natural position so that the breathing is unrestricted. The following pose will help you to relax properly.

Corpse Pose

Sit comfortably on the floor with your knees bent and your feet flat on the floor. Place your hands on the floor, bend your elbows and allow your upper body to drop gently back, supporting yourself with your hands, forearms and elbows.

Sliding your hands forwards, roll gently through your spine down onto the floor so that you are lying flat with your knees still bent.

Slide your feet forward and press the backs of your knees and legs into the floor.

Separate your arms and legs a few inches and turn them outwards. Do not let them flop.

Shut your eyes and slow your breathing until it reaches a regular, deep rhythm.

Starting with your toes, begin to relax each part of your body in turn, working from your toes to your feet to your ankles and so on. If some part seems particularly tense then gently contract it before allowing the muscles to relax.

Try to let any distracting thoughts simply drift through your head, letting them go with each out-breath.

Once your body is totally relaxed, enjoy the sensation for a few minutes or as long as you need before gently coming to sitting and then to standing.

Try to keep that feeling of relaxation with you as you carry on with your session or day.

Simple Yoga Session

The following yoga session is based upon the particularly gentle form called Sivananda yoga and is suitable for complete beginners as well as for more experienced yoga practitioners.

Remember to take extra care if you suffer from any injury or lower back pain, consulting a health professional if necessary before you undertake these exercises.

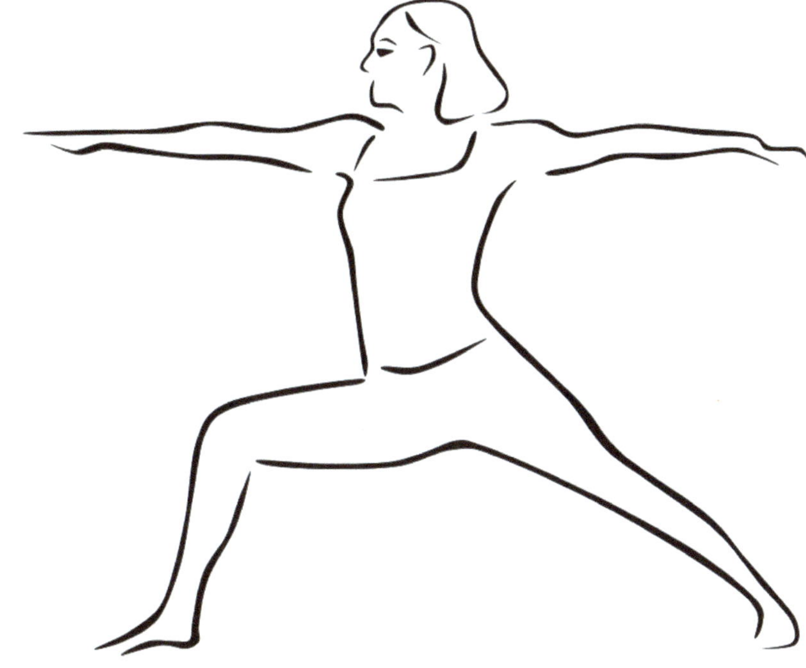

The Cleansing Breath

This exercise is also known as Kapalabhati which means 'shining skull' and it is designed to cleanse the respiratory system, feed oxygen to the lungs and drain the sinuses.

It also eliminates excess carbon dioxide from the body, purifying the blood and increasing prana.

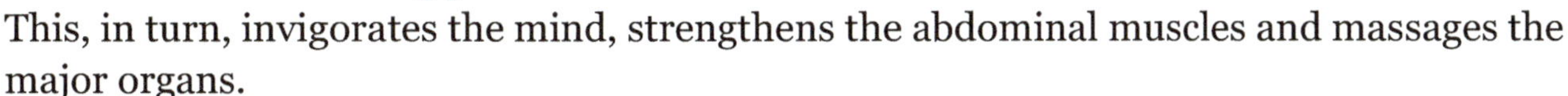

This, in turn, invigorates the mind, strengthens the abdominal muscles and massages the major organs.

Sit tall and comfortably with your back as straight as possible. Try to relax your abdominal muscles as you breathe freely.

Inhale gently through the nose, allowing your lungs and abdomen to expand. It may help to imagine both of these as balloons filling with air.

Now exhale sharply through your nose, pulling in your abdominal muscles as you do so and pushing the air out of your lungs.

Do this 10 times and then rest.

Yoga – The Secret to Stress-Free Living

Practice this morning and evening. Start by exhaling once per second, building up so that you are exhaling twice per second and increasing from 10 breaths to 20 and then 30 and so on until you can perform 120 exhalations in each session. Don't worry if this takes some practice!

Alternate Nostril Breathing

This exercise strengthens and purifies the lungs while also increasing prana intake.

Sit tall and as straight as possible on the floor and breathe freely. Curl the index and middle finger of your right hand into your palm so that you can use your thumb and fourth finger either side of your nose to close each nostril in turn.

Breathe in through both nostrils.

Using your right hand as described in step one, close your right nostril with your right thumb and breathe out through your left nostril on a count of four.

Now breathe in through your left nostril on a count of four.

Close your left nostril with the fourth finger of your right hand, breathing out through your right nostril to a count of four.

Breathe in through the right nostril to a count of four.

Close the right nostril and breathe out through the left nostril to a count of four.

Breathe in through the left nostril to a count of four.

Release your right nostril and exhale on a long, slow out-breath.

It can take some time to get used to this breathing technique but persevere and try to build up the length and depth of the inhalations and the exhalations.

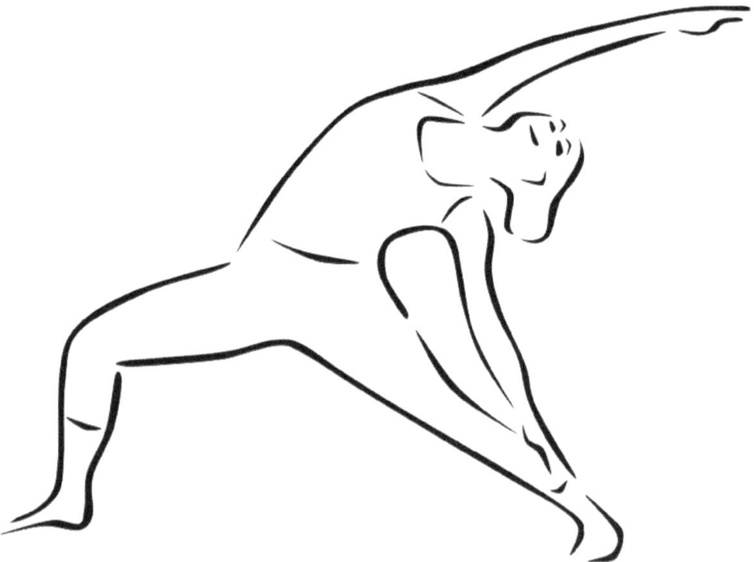

Yoga – The Secret to Stress-Free Living

Asanas

This sequence consists of 12 movements which can be practised by anyone of any age.

Perform them once through at first, building up until you can do them 15 times in five minutes.

Stand tall in the Mountain posture, Tadasana, you learned in the warm-up section, with your feet together. Inhale deeply, exhale and place your hands in prayer position at chest height.

On a long inhalation, stretch your arms up over your head, arching your spine so you are leaning backwards and gazing up.

On your exhalation, fold into a forward bend with your head leading, hands placed either side of your feet.

Inhale and stretch your left foot backwards, placing the left knee on the floor. Look up without straining the neck or chin.

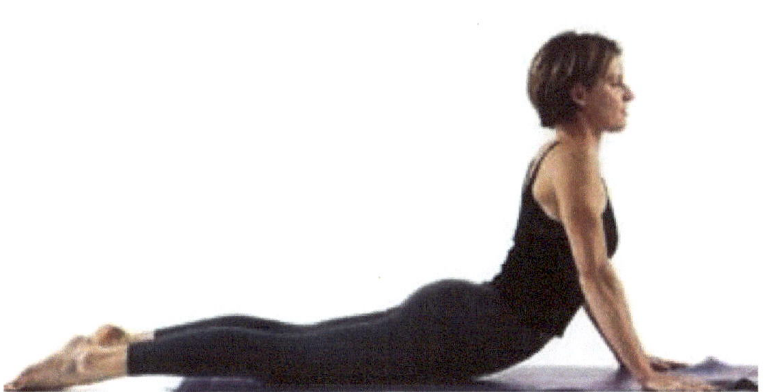

Now bring your right leg back and, holding your breath, extend into a push-up position with both legs straight and in line from shoulders to hips to heels, balancing on your curled-in toes.

Exhale and drop your knees to the floor, lowering your chest to the floor between your hands as you bend your arms. Drop your chin or forehead to the floor, depending on what feels more comfortable for you. Do not strain your neck.

On an inhalation, slide forwards, push up on your hands and arms so that they are nearly straight and arch your spine into Cobra posture, looking up. Your legs and feet remain stretched out on the floor, toes pointed.

Yoga – The Secret to Stress-Free Living

On an exhalation, push your hips up and back so that you form the downward facing triangular shape known as downward dog. Your legs should be as straight as possible and you should be gazing at the floor.

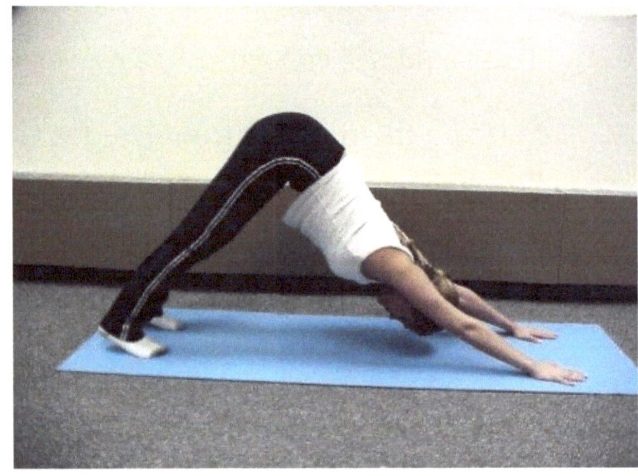

Try to stretch your heels down so that your feet are flat on the floor although you may find this difficult at first. Do not force this stretch.

Inhale and slide your right foot forwards, bending it at the knee and placing it between your hands. Drop your left knee to the floor with the left leg still stretching back. Look up without straining chin or neck.

Exhale and move the left foot forward to join the right foot. Fold yourself over your bent knees and straighten into a standing forward bend, head to knees.

Inhale and stretch your arms, swinging them so you come back to standing with arms stretched backwards, back arched and gaze upwards as you did in step two.

Exhale and let your arms fall gently to your sides. Relax.

This sequence tones and strengthens your entire system. By synchronizing your breath with your movements, you exercise all your muscles while improving blood flow and gently increasing heart rate.

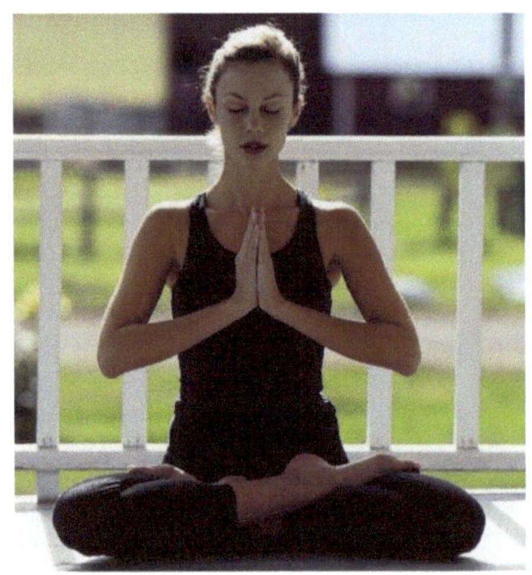

Savasana

Practice the Corpse pose as you were taught in the warm-up sequence. This eases out body and mind as you assimilate the benefits of your asana practice. You may like to add a mantra while relaxing and can choose from one of the suggestions given earlier in this book.

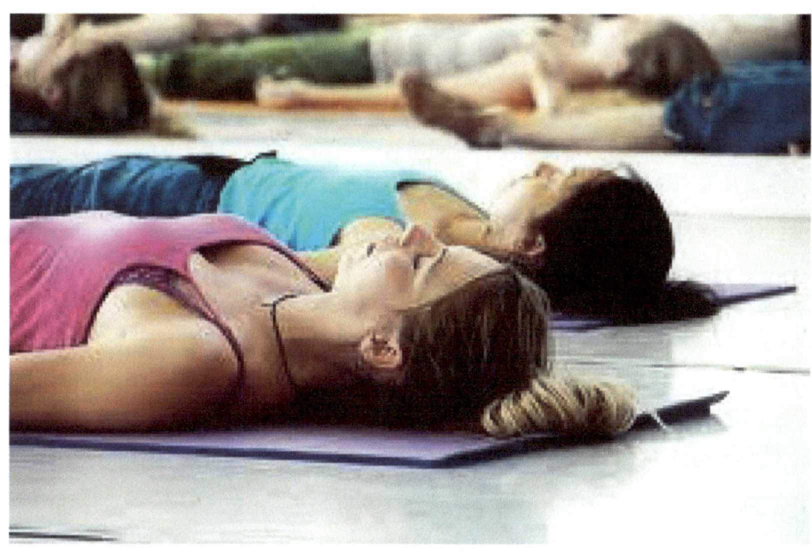

Conclusion

Yoga is not only an excellent system for mind and body, it is a way to clear your mind and lift your mood so that you can adopt a more positive attitude to life.

By practicing yoga, you learn to open your heart which naturally increases your sense of gratitude for all that you have and all the life has to offer.

Gratitude is central to yoga and to positivity. It is also well known as an antidote to the depression and stress that afflict so many people in our modern, hectic world.

Practiced yogis look on gratitude as a waking meditation and as something we must remind ourselves to do every day.

If you take time every day to notice all the good things in your life you will begin to find that more and more of them appear.

One of those good things should, of course, be yoga – the ancient system that has given us so much over the centuries and continues to sustain and nourish us with its unique form of life-enhancing practice.

Why not make this the day you begin to give yourself the gift of yoga?

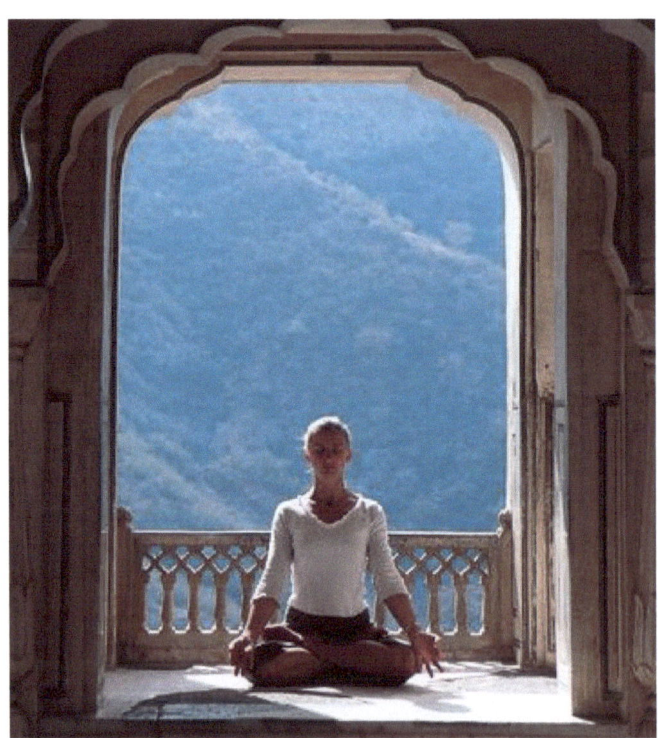

Recommended Resources

https://www.amazon.com/gp/product/1544837364

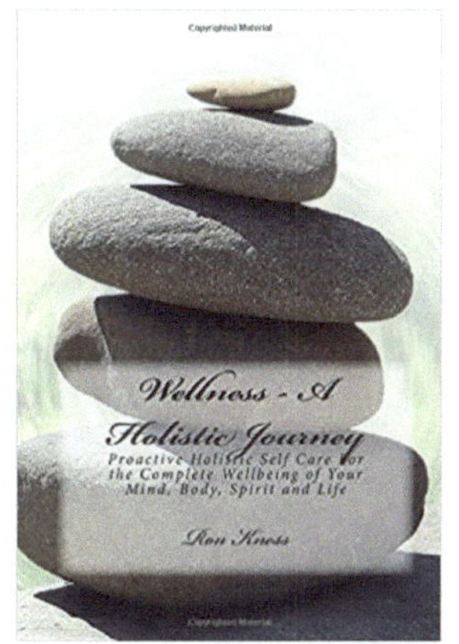

Wellness - A Holistic Journey: Proactive Holistic Self Care For the Complete Wellbeing of Your Mind, Body, Spirit and Life

Incredibly, you have this amazing healing power inside yourself, all you must do is follow the proper path with the right information to create an overall healthy state of being.

By attaining ultimate wellbeing holistically, we are allowing ourselves to express our full capacity as human beings, and we are choosing to walk as warriors of light and positive influence through a world that is often cold and dark…

https://www.amazon.com/gp/product/1535511370

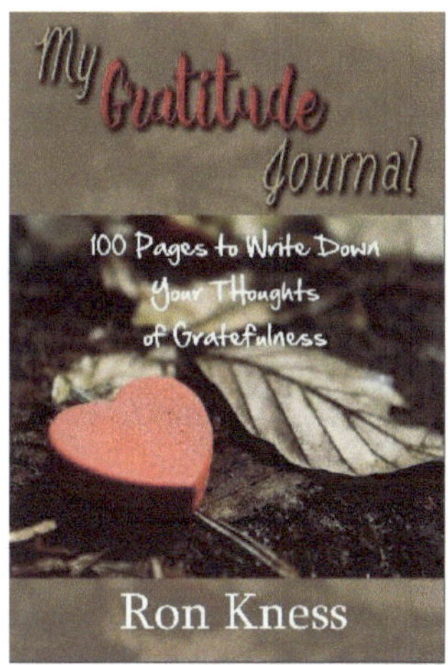

My Gratitude Journal: 100 Pages to Write Down What You Are Grateful for in Your Life

When you express or feel gratitude, you're acknowledging that there is good in your life, in you, in the world and all around you. With the way things are in the world right now, we can all use acknowledge of something good! Feeling grateful changes how you feel inside. It is an easy way to reduce stress in your life.

It's easy to let the negative thoughts, words, situations, events, and actions in the world take over your heart and mind. Many in society seem to focus on the negative; we know the media does. It's on the news, in magazines and newspapers, and it may be the general tone of the conversations you encounter during the day. Yet, the simple emotion and expression of gratitude diminishes all of that negativity in a powerful way.

Make this journal your "happy place" where you can go and record thoughts of positivity to overcome the negativeness all around you in your life right now. You will feel better in the end.

https://www.amazon.com/gp/product/1543029418

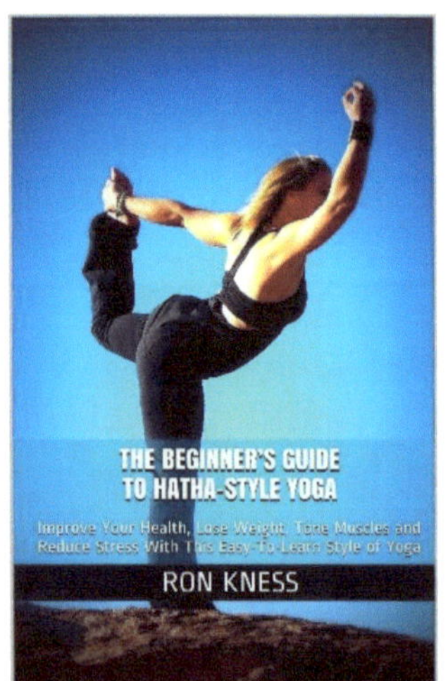

The Beginner's Guide to Hatha-Style Yoga: Improve Your Health, Lose Weight, Tone Muscles and Reduce Stress With This Easy-To-Learn Style of Yoga

Based on these exciting teachings, you will learn about all the dramatic benefits of doing Hatha yoga like improved health, weight loss, muscle toning and reducing stress, along with improved flexibility and balance. This book is built around a very clear, concept: learn yoga and reap the benefits from doing this style of yoga - Hatha.

It's not just about learning how to do this easy-to-learn style of yoga. Having great overall health is linked to being in charge and making smart healthy lifestyle decisions. This is because learning how to do any style of yoga should be part of any healthy lifestyle. In this book, we look at all of the ways you can improve your own overall health, starting with deciding to learn the poses and practice yoga.

This book will also look at the many other steps that can be taken to support this goal, like viewing the suggested videos of poses used in Hatha yoga depending on the health benefit you want to gain. The choices you make about joining a Hatha yoga class or learning it by yourself and doing it at home has a great impact on your overall health.

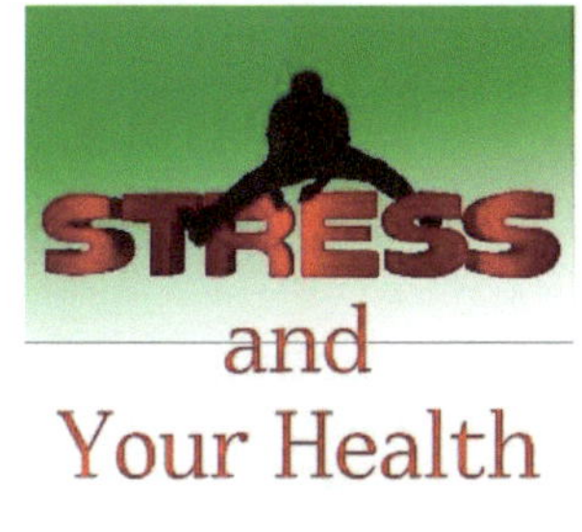

Stress and Your Health: Recognize the Signs, Symptoms and Adverse Effects Over Time

While the word "stress" has many different meanings, as discussed in this publication it refers to the health condition which is all but endemic in modern society. The human body, mind and all its sub-systems developed to deal with the challenges of much more primitive circumstances than we live in now.

Our rapid-response "fight or flight" response system enabled our species to outperform and out-think our way past all others. Collectively our incredible brains have allowed us to live today in a manner that does not require us to engage in the type of activities that made our stress hormones a major asset.

Unfortunately, our physiology has not kept pace with our intellectual development and there is no magic switch to turn off or at least turn down our survival responses.

Today, in civilized societies, we encounter a different manner of struggles and challenges. Even though these situations may not actually be life or death in nature, because of the emotion we attach to our various actions, our minds perceive them as such, and react accordingly.

For many or most people, their bodies and mind are in a constant state of heightened anxiety due to the continually elevated levels of stress hormones in their system. This is chronic stress and its symptoms are broad, varied and can ultimately even be fatal.

We are taught so many things that enable us to live in a social environment with our fellow humans, but too many of us lack knowledge of how to deal with the pressure and stress this can apply.

Inability to deal with the causes of stress leads to increased stress and inability to deal with the symptoms of stress can make life seem not worth living. This publication details some of the signs and symptoms of chronic stress and their damaging effects on our minds and bodies. If you feel stress is negatively impacting your life, make changes by reducing the causes, or learn to cope with them more appropriately to lessen the impact on you.

About the Author

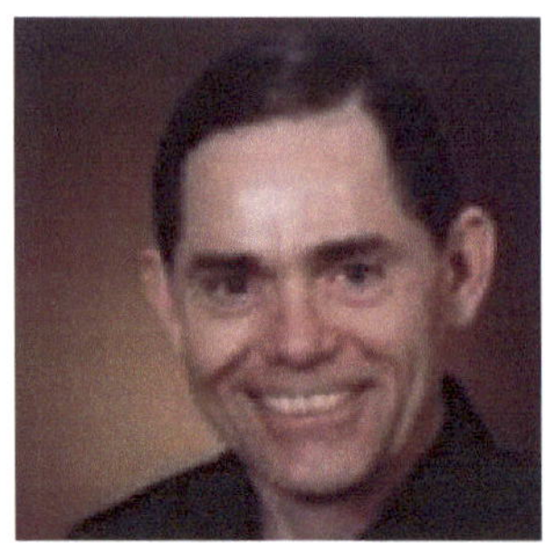

I have published numerous books on Amazon and other publishing platforms.

While most of my books are on health and fitness in general, as I age (now 65) at the time of this writing) my topics of interest are geared toward aging baby boomers and older.

Besides my own writing, I also ghostwrite ebooks, books, reports, articles, blogs and do Kindle conversions for clients on a variety of topics.

Today my wife and I are retired from our careers and live in San Tan Valley, AZ. I now write as a retirement business where you'll find me happily sitting in my office typing away on my laptop as I work on my next book or ghostwriting project . . . that is if we are not traveling on a cruise ship - our new-found mode of travel.